New Hearts, New Lives

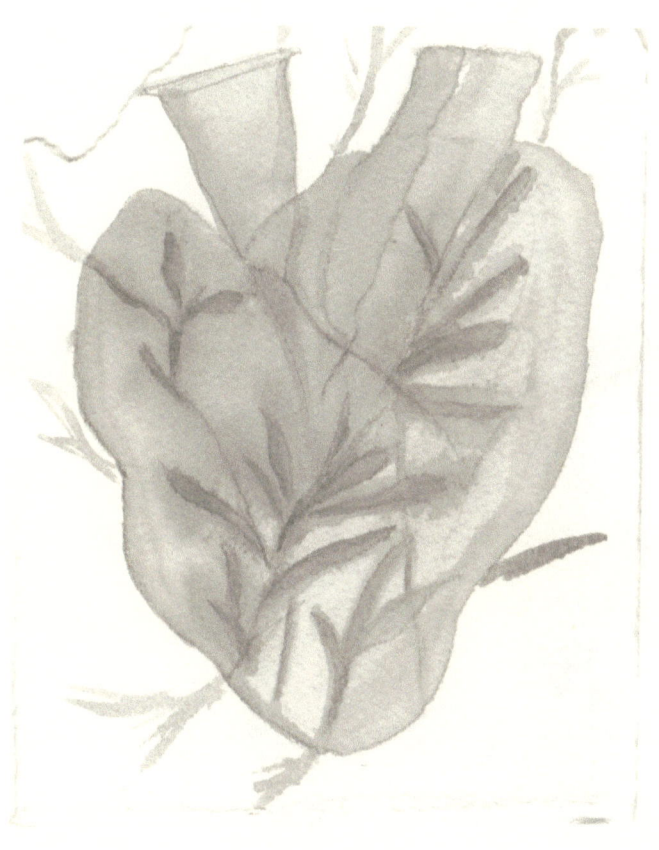

New Hearts, New Lives

Richard D. Lueker, M.D.

Christopher J. Lueker-Ritter, Ph.D.

Lulu

2018

First Printing: 2017. Second Printing: 2018.

ISBN 978-1-387-40412-4

Lulu Press, Inc.
627 Davis Drive Suite 300
Morrisville, NC 27560

Contents

Acknowledgements

The authors would like to thank all of the people we interviewed for this book, whose stories of suffering and rehabilitating from heart disease illustrate the full range of human response to adversity. Surviving heart disease was an inspiring act of resilience; sharing your stories was an inspiring act of generosity.

We would also like to thank our wives, Meg and Alison, without whose support and encouragement this book would not exist.

Preface

Christopher J. Ritter, Ph.D.

Many people can't wait to retire from the toil of their career, but my father-in-law was not one of them. Dick Lueker sincerely loved helping people heal, and loved working with his staff of dedicated caregivers at New Heart Cardiac Rehabilitation. So he didn't even begin winding down his work at New Heart until he approached 80; and even then, he kept working, downloading his 50 years of knowledge and experience into what would become this book.

Dick wasn't writing a memoir, though; this was no act of ego. When he approached me for help with his manuscript, I asked him what he wanted the book to do for its readers. He responded with a story.

Many years ago, Dick was addressing a new cohort of patients at New Heart, showing them around the facility, explaining how their rehabilitation process would work. Spontaneously, one of his experienced patients, who was exercising nearby, walked over to the group of newbies and started telling them his own story. Dick, ever-attendant to other people's inspiration, stopped his spiel and listened to the man. He also watched the newbies as they listened, noticing that they paid greater attention to this peer's story than they had to his doctorly lecture. They were rapt; their eyes shone. When Dick thought about interjecting something, he heard an inner voice say, "Be quiet. They need to hear from someone like them." Since he is also ever-attendant to divine inspiration, he heeded that voice. And he remembered it forever.

Dick understood that while patients get information and guidance from healthcare professionals, they get comfort and inspiration from people like themselves. So what he really wanted this book to do was let heart disease survivors speak to other heart disease survivors. It is our hope that someone contemplating cardiac rehabilitation will be inspired to start, that someone undergoing rehab will be inspired to continue, and that someone completing rehab will be inspired to share his or her story.

Introduction

Richard D. Lueker, M.D.

An epidemic surging through the United States? Were you aware? Could it possibly be true?

The United States has been in a "silent" growing epidemic for the past several decades. Silent because we, the people, are unaware. It is hard to imagine, but it is true. We would like to believe that Americans are strong and healthy. We believe that we are the best and the strongest, and we would like to think of ourselves as invincible. We have the best of everything, and therefore we must have the best health as well. We have all heard information that heart disease has been turning a corner during the last 10-15 years. Deaths from heart disease are being reduced. Public health reports indicate that early deaths from heart disease are on the decline. Coronary care units, coronary angioplasty, and heart surgery have reduced death rates from this disease. Unfortunately, such is not the case.

Health experts indicate that we are in the midst of an epidemic that may threaten to change our way of life as a society. We are not as strong or as healthy as we once were, "once upon a time." Over the years, subtle changes have occurred, changes in our lifestyles that threaten to harm us, individually and collectively. We don't see people falling over the streets, but year after year the heart disease epidemic continues to grow, and it may influence and even bankrupt our country — physically, socially, and even economically —

if we don't change course. Heart disease is still the #1 disease in our country. Scientists have speculated that within a decade, heart disease will be the #1 illness throughout the world, even eclipsing AIDS. Experts predict that within the next 10 years we will have more heart disease in the United States than the total number of people living in Canada. Life expectancy for citizens in the USA — approximately 70-75 years — ranks approximately 30th in the world. Life expectancy in European countries is higher than in the USA. In Japan, life expectancy for men and women is nearly 85 years. Researchers also indicate that because of the epidemic of heart disease, children born after the year 2000 will not live as long as their parents.

The work of Dr. Dee Edington at the University of Michigan provides an extra cost — a monetary cost. Edington has stated that increasing numbers of health risk factors are associated with greater monetary costs for our society. In other words, more people with increasing risks are costing themselves and the rest of us more and more. Spending more and more on the costs of healthcare will leave less and less for some of the important things we need to do for our society, like building schools, improving highways and bridges and more. The wider and wider spread of poor health may break our bank.

These are shocking revelations. How could they be true?

True, we have wonderful hospitals, well established coronary care units, sophisticated obstetrical and delivery units, skilled surgical and interventional specialists. We have a wonderful disease care system in the United States. (Notice the subtly different phrase — I said "disease care system," not "health care system.") We do an excellent job caring for people when they get sick, but we do not do a good job preventing the disease from occurring in the first place. This is of great concern to our society, and all health care experts agree.

How so you might say? The habits that lead to heart disease and many other diseases have become, to a large extent, a way of life for the average American:

We eat too much.

We exercise too little.

We work too hard.

We unwind with drugs and alcohol.

These are some of the reasons that heart disease continues to increase in our country, but the primary factors are obesity and diabetes. These risk factors have been studied by researchers for many years.

The following maps of the United States show the increase in the levels of obesity and diabetes from 1994 to 2009. Notice how each map gets darker, perhaps as an omen, over time.

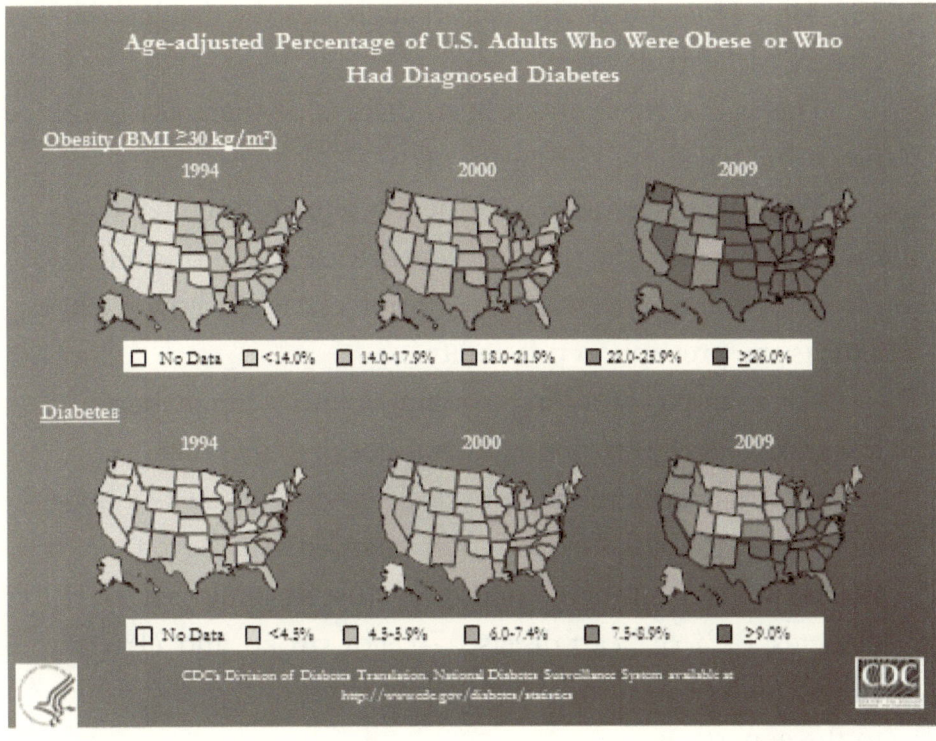

These risk factors and their frequency have been steadily increasing in our society. The number of people with risk factors is growing. So the incidence of heart disease continues to increase.

These risk factors have a multiplying effect: the more risk factors a person has, the greater his or her likelihood of developing disease. Also, more risk factors result in heart disease earlier in life. This was dramatically expressed in an article by Dr. Salim Yousuf, who summarized the significance of the increased number of risk factors related to heart disease. If a person has only one risk factor, the risk of heart disease increases by twofold; if a person has 3 risk factors, the risk goes up 42-fold; at 6 risk factors, the danger increases 182-fold. Thus, more risk factors increases the danger, the chance of heart disease.

This is bad news about heart disease. Is there any good news that we should be aware of?

Yes, there is good news. There is a great potential to dramatically alter the onset of this disease, or to prevent it. How? By the way we take care of ourselves and how we live. This is the prevention possibility.

For example, stopping smoking, controlling diabetes, lowering blood pressure, reducing obesity, lowering cholesterol and increasing physical activity can make a huge difference. Remarkably, low-cost interventions have the highest impact on these conditions. Just imagine that 91 % of diabetes, 82% of heart disease, 70% of stroke, and 71% of colon cancer can be avoided with lifestyle changes according to the experts.

This is not about different treatments, different medications, or greater medical and surgical advances. It is about how we live, how we spend our time, how we become more active. It's also about our emotions — joy, fear, anger, and even forgiveness — and how they affect our lives. Medical experts indicate that if we pay more attention to our physical and mental health, such attention may play a major role in our happiness and longevity.

Victory after a heart attack? Impossible! Yes it is possible. Even after heart disease strikes, it is possible to push it back.

Here are stories of men and women who suffered from heart attacks or heart surgery or both, and are now living victorious lives. They have suffered through the fears and anxieties in and out of the hospital. They have been in coronary care units and on operating tables, and they have experienced all of the emotional shocks and fears that you and your loved ones have experienced. They have been down, discouraged, depressed, and anxious about the future of their lives. However, all these folks made a significant decision to improve their health. They are doing all the things they want to do, not worrying that their "heart" will not tolerate their new lifestyle.

I have had the experience of working with each of these people, and I have watched them as they have pushed back and fought against heart disease. We have worked with them, coached them and encouraged them. Many have made amazing changes in their health and in their lives.

What kinds of changes? They have pushed and stretched themselves not only to regain their health but also, in the in the process, to become stronger and healthier than they had ever been. They have proven that it is possible that people may improve their health and fitness by steady effort and training. Their stories are encouraging because they have demonstrated that a person's health, strength and potential may be improved by physical training like an athlete. The stories have dramatized and proven that people may improve even as they age, even though they may have had major health problems including heart attacks and surgery. These individuals tested their limits and expanded their potential. These people are Overcomers.

One of these Overcomers, Durand, rode a 55-mile bike race over two 10,000-foot passes within 11 months of suffering a major heart attack. Another, Rudy, hiked through the California mountains for over 10 days with a 50-pound backpack just one year after he had a heart attack.

Other stories in this book are less dramatic but are still significant. Pamela has lost 74 pounds in the course of her recovery, and has learned profound lessons about giving care to herself as well as to her family. Helen has learned about nutrition, exercise, and mindfulness as she recovers from a heart attack whose causes are still murky. David experienced divine encouragement in the course of his recovery, which ultimately complemented his rational worldview.

Other stories here illustrate lessons about one's attitude towards hereditary heart disease. Both Gregg and Francis have drawn upon their faith in order to approach their disease without suffering from it.

These seven people are a tiny fraction of the heart disease survivors that have worked with New Heart Cardiac Rehabilitation. We have observed remarkable physical achievements in many of those who have suffered heart attacks and/or heart surgery but didn't give up and fought back. Many folks, perhaps just like you, made a decision not to give up but to rejoin the human race, perhaps literally. They have all said, "I don't want to re-experience heart disease, and I will do whatever it takes to build a strong, healthy body and beat this heart trouble."

It's helpful for people who have recently been affected by heart disease to learn firsthand from those who have experienced heart disease and recovered. It is our hope that this will give you courage, so that you may also be an Overcomer.

Ultimately, all of these stories are about hope. Not hope that is impossible, but hope that is real and that has been achieved in the hearts of many people we will describe in these next pages. To quote Proverbs 13:12, "Hope deferred makes the heart sick, but a longing fulfilled is a tree of life."

We hope that these stories may give you encouragement and hope, so that you can join the people in this book in the club of heart disease survivors. May this give you inspiration and courage to discover the glorious life that awaits you, even after a heart attack.

1.   The Self-Denier

Editors' introduction

In many ways, "Pamela" is the stereotypical American heart attack victim: a type-A personality who willfully charged through stress, ignored her body, and contracted heart disease. However, as her story shows, she was motivated not by selfishness but by selflessness.

Pamela's story

Put simply, I got heart disease because I was caring for others and neglecting myself.

In my 30s, I was active and healthy, but life piled stress upon me, and I didn't respond healthily to it. My father developed Alzheimer's when I was 32. By the time I was 35, I held a high-pressure job as a professional fundraiser. When I was 40, I adopted a child with mental illness. My dad passed that year, and my mom was aging quickly. I was doing the woman-in-the-middle-of-the-sandwich thing.

As you can imagine, all the caregiving I was doing was making my blood pressure rise: it was consistently above normal, like 145/110.[i] I started taking the blood pressure drug lisprinil at a low dose, and my primary physician suggested that I take a statin.[ii] But she wasn't very adamant about it, so her mild warnings didn't shake me out of denial about my health.

Denial infected every element of my lifestyle. I dieted like the fast-paced American I was: I ate out sometimes three times a day, and snacked on sweets at night. (I'm still addicted to bread!) I didn't treat good food like a treat; I treated it like an everyday occurrence. And I didn't do anything to burn off all those calories. I was a member of a gym, but member was the operative word. I didn't do any exercise, didn't do any meditation; I just led a sedentary life. So my weight kept climbing, along with my cholesterol.

Heart disease hit me like it's hit a lot of women I've met: minor warning signs (very tired and a dull ache behind my sternum), plus an overriding feeling of doom. I knew there was something really wrong with me, but I couldn't' tell really what it was.

I went to urgent care first. This was both the wrong move and the right move: they could only take an EKG and blood work, but they realized that my situation was serious and put me on an ambulance for the hospital. That's where I had my heart attack — in the ambulance!

My experience at the hospital was mixed. The first doctor I met there had to stop talking to me when he found out he wasn't in my insurance network. But I eventually got helped by the right people, and they put a big stent in my main coronary artery.[iii] Fortunately, I didn't suffer any muscle-tissue death in my heart, even though it was ischemic.[iv]

I realized that I had to change my life — and quickly — but the recovery was tough for the first six months. I felt tons of anxiety; I kept thinking, "Will the stent really work?" I mean every little feeling — everything — scared me.[v] And it was hard to capture time for exercise.

Fortunately, I had great guidance at New Heart. I loved it there, because I realized that it's a family of people. Dr. Lueker helped me recognize the difference between serious chest pain and a pulled muscle. A therapist helped me see how I had been bottling everything up, and helped me learn to shift stress away from myself. Through New Heart's Integrative Wellness classes, I discovered mindfulness: mindful eating, mindful work, mind-body stress relief. I felt very cared for by the New Heart staff, and that helped me through my fear. I also met a lot of other women in rehabilitation that were embracing change. The men talked like their bodies were cars — "I got the piece fixed, I got a new thing here, I'm fine." They were still eating gloppy stuff, red meat, fried stuff. But the women were scared to death, and they took rehabilitation more earnestly.

My recovery was gradual at first — I could only exercise for a minute or two at a time. But I was serious about it. I started exercising 5-6 days a week, walking 7,000-10,000 steps a day. I stopped drinking caffeine and eating sugar. I went back to Weight Watchers with a very specific goal in mind.

I started feeling better within a couple weeks of my heart attack, but people have told me it took me about six to nine months to get back to who I am, personality-wise. Getting back to being me was what gave me hope every day.

It's been two and a half years since my heart attack, and according to my husband, I am back. In July 2016, I met my goal: a 74-pound total weight loss. But I'm also better because things roll off of me a lot easier.

Getting over a heart attack is a package of things. I meditate twice a day for 20 minutes — in the morning, and just before bed — and sometimes also in the car, with my eyes open. I like Judy Grossel's guided meditation tapes, because her voice doesn't grate on my ears. Mindfulness has been the key, especially around the eating. Mostly, mindfulness has helped me learn not to hold onto things, because I know what they're going to do to me if I do. I've tried to remove myself from toxic people; and if even my friends are stressing me out, they know that I'm now likely to walk away from them. I've quit a couple of volunteer jobs after realizing that they were too stressful. I only do stuff that I like now. (I know this is a luxury; when you're working full time, you can't always make those choices.) I'm still working on my Ph.D. — this is a bucket list thing for me — but I recently told my committee that I needed to slow down at it. To give it up would be very hard, but I'm fully prepared to do so if it gets too stressful. I don't want to quit before I get the brass ring, but the heart attack made me realize that I could be gone in a second.

Mindfulness has also taught me to appreciate the measurable results of my recovery, like positive tests and negative pounds. I'm listening now, and I'm asking a lot of questions. I still experience worry — like during a recent trip, when I had to go through airport metal detectors, and spent a lot of time on my feet — but I've noticed that I've turned a corner with the fear. It was gradual, but I see it now.

I'm really outgoing, I'm a big personality, so now I feel compelled to warn people that are where I used to be. All these people walking around with obesity problems, they never think they're gonna pay a price for that. I would tell them to take their health really seriously. If you're uncomfortable with your provider, do something about it. If you gain back time — through retiring, or quitting a volunteer thing, or losing a parent you were caring for, or emptying your nest when your kid moves out — don't fill it up with junk. Fill it up with something that's meaningful, that benefits you. Take back your time. Live your life, and don't be scared. [vi]

2. The Grateful Sufferer

Editors' introduction

The first thing one notices about Gregg Peevy is that he is self-effacing. He apologizes throughout the interview — for talking for a long time (he's an excellent interviewee, needing little prompting), for his notes on his illness "not being better" (they're extensive and meticulous), for "not wanting to come off as a religious nut" (he doesn't: his faith has clearly kept him sane through his long ordeal).

The second thing one notices is that Gregg seems exhausted but happy. He speaks in a raspy voice that's sometimes little more than a whisper, as if he is profoundly tired. Which makes sense as his story unfolds: he's spent the last eleven years battling heart disease, his former life as an engineer devolving into the life of a perpetual patient. But he smiles a lot, his eyes crinkling, as he recalls the support he's found from his wife, his church, and his fellow heart disease survivors. Throughout our interview, he repeatedly expresses gratitude for his trial. "I wouldn't want to do it again, that's for sure," he says, "but on one hand, I'm thankful for it. You see that people love you and care for you. On one hand, it was terrible; on the other hand, it was wonderful."

Gregg's story is full of dichotomies like this, beginning with his initial illness.

Gregg's story

In 2001, at age 41, I was getting a routine physical, and the doctor told me he was concerned about the sound of my heart. I was used to hearing doctors say this, because I'd had a heart murmur[vii] my entire life. Besides, I felt completely healthy. But the doctor insisted that something else was wrong: I had a prolapsed mitral valve,[viii] which had caused severe mitral valve regurgitation with cardiomyopathy,[ix] and I needed to have it repaired within three months to delay or stop the cardiomyopathy and heart failure. It was very shocking that I would need heart surgery in three months, because I felt fine outwardly.

My first intervention was a mitral valve repair with a Delran ring.[x] The surgery was performed at Presbyterian Hospital in Albuquerque, NM.

And here my troubles really began.

The first surgery successfully repaired my mitral valve, but it also caused an arrhythmia[xi] in my heart as a side effect. I had to take medications to counteract the arrhythmia, but the medications made me feel sluggish. Ironically, the medications that were required to keep me alive put a damper on my activities. But I was in denial — I would kinda buck at things: I kept rollerblading, as I had always done, and I pushed my doctors to decrease the medications as much as possible.

Two years later, I had two events where I thought I was going to pass out. The first was at home; the second was the next day at work, which concluded with an ambulance ride to the hospital. However, the emergency room doctors were not able to diagnose the problem, since I felt better once I arrived there. They set up an appointment with my cardiologist for two days later.

I arrived at my appointment after I had just helped a friend move some luggage, the exertion of which had made me feel extremely run-down, as if I could hardly move. When I arrived at the cardiologist's office, the front desk assistants said, "Gregg, you don't look well," and I admitted that I didn't. So they sent me back to a room so the nurses could take an EKG. The nurse took the EKG and ran to get the doctor, who rushed in and told me that I was having an episode of ventricular tachycardia[xii] because my heart rate was 237 beats per minute. The cardiologist took my phone and called my wife to inform her that she was rushing me to the hospital to deal with the tachycardia. There, the cardiologist put me on an even stronger anti-arrhythmia drug. This drug started exacerbating other health problems, like hemorrhoids.

After another two years, in 2005, I negotiated with my cardiologist to be put on a less-strong anti-arrhythmia drug, which had fewer side effects, with the caveat that I would get an Implanted Cardio Defibrillator (ICD).[xiii] The ICD would shock my heart when it detected a sustained potential life-threatening arrhythmia. The ICD would start with a low level of shock, but that felt like putting my hand on an electrical wire. This happened on two occasions, seemingly without warning, since the ICD would trigger before I even felt anything. Fortunately, it never had to shock me at the higher levels.

Also in 2005, my father died of heart failure. Both of my parents, it turned out, had mitral valve problems, so my own heart problems were unavoidable.

However, I was still in this denial mode, where I would try to reduce my medications down to the lowest level so I would feel more energetic. My relationship with most of my doctors contributed to this denial: their office visit times were limited, and I interpreted their hurried, brusque conversations like, "Oh, things must not be that big a deal because they're not having serious talks with me." We just didn't spend enough time together for them to recognize that I was in denial.

At the same time, I did start addressing my heart health more consciously, starting cardiac rehabilitation at New Heart in 2005. I liked it, because Dr. Lueker would talk to me and give me the time I needed (more time than a normal doctor's office visit). He educated me on my heart condition and the medications I was taking, and he introduced me to others with serious heart problems. Dr. Lueker became my friend and a big encouragement to me.

My condition was stable for the next three and a half years, until 2009. In the spring, I began to notice I had swelling in my ankles and legs: I could push my finger into my ankle and form a dent that wouldn't go away.[xiv] In the summer, I went on a walk with my wife at the end of a stressful day at work and couldn't keep up with her. I felt short of breath and thought I was having an asthma attack, which I'd had as a kid. I tried my albuterol inhaler, but my shortness of breath and wheezing did not improve. By now, trips to the emergency room were becoming so routine that I told my wife to stay home.

I checked into the emergency room thinking I just had asthma problems, not having a clue that I was having serious heart problems. The emergency room personnel believed my theory about the asthma, triaged me with an intravenous port in my arm, and put me back in the waiting room. As I was sitting in the waiting room with an IV in my arm, two young women were sitting nearby in wheelchairs crying in pain, and another man was lying on the floor crying out with stomach pain. There was a movie on the television about the life of Michael Jackson in memorial of his recent death. I thought, "I am in Hell. I am not in that bad of shape. I would leave this emergency room but I have this IV port in my arm." It is a good thing I stayed: eventually, the nurses came and performed an EKG and an echocardiogram. The doctors determined that I had congestive heart failure. xv

I wound up spending the next seven days in the hospital, having all the fluid that was backed up in my lungs drained out of me and being put on a new regimen of heart failure medications, which did improve my ejection fraction. My cardiologist recommended that I retire — stress at work had been getting to me, the heart problems had been going on for eight years, and the future looked uncertain. At the same time, a young new doctor that was replacing my current cardiologist suggested I might need a heart transplant. I could not fathom that yet.

I took the doctor's advice and retired, feeling very grateful for every extra day. But my heart failure continued, along with various interventions. I had atrial fibrillation[xvi] and flutter in December of 2010, so I underwent a heart ablation (a-fib)[xvii] in May of 2011. But I developed ventricular tachycardia, [xviii] so I had another ablation in December of 2011. By the beginning of 2012, after so many interventions on a heart that just kept failing, I began to consider getting a transplant.[xix]

A friend from work who'd also had heart failure introduced me to Intermountain Medical Center (IMC) in Utah, which had a good record on transplants. So my wife and I flew to Salt Lake City for a heart transplant evaluation.[xx] I was still in denial, I remember — I thought I was just having an office visit — but the IMC doctors admitted me to the hospital for a battery of tests that took a week. During the evaluation the doctors removed my old ICD and replaced it with a biventricular (BiV) ICD[xxi] in an attempt to synchronize my heart chamber function in order to keep me going until my heart transplant. I passed the tests and got on IMC's transplant list, but since I have O+ blood type, I was told that my wait might be longer than usual. The doctors told me to wait six months before moving to Utah.

However, the BiV ICD did not benefit my heart that much, and I had to unexpectedly return to Utah after a month and a half. My wife and I packed two bags and flew to Utah, not knowing that it would be a year and half before we could return home. When I arrived at IMC, I was immediately admitted into the Intensive Care Unit. I was put on a dobutamine IV drip.[xxii] But the doctors said that I was now on a "slippery slope" and recommended I have a left ventricular assist device (LVAD)[xxiii] installed to take over some of the function of my deteriorating heart and keep me alive until the transplant. The LVAD horrified me initially — it meant being constantly hooked up to a machine that was attached to my heart to circulate my blood, controlled through a drive-line that was connected percutaneously through my abdomen to a controller I would have to wear around my waist — but I agreed to it, because it also meant that I'd get to be at the very top of the transplant list for a month.

While I was recovering for a month in the hospital from the LVAD surgery, my wife made a quick trip back to Albuquerque to pick up a laptop from her employer so she could telecommute from Salt Lake City and keep her job. Also during this time, my friends from church packed up my house in Albuquerque so a church family could move in and house-sit during the time that I and my wife would be away. The packed items from my house were put in a moving van, which my friends then drove, along with one of my vehicles, to Utah, and unpacked them in my new apartment.

For the next seven months, my wife and I lived in an apartment in Salt Lake City, very near the hospital, where I went three times a week. It was rough adapting to the LVAD for the first three months. I was on blood thinners, which made me bleed everywhere.[xxiv] But over time, I got feeling better and stronger. Eventually, I was able to drive, visit friends, attend church meetings, and go to the mountains surrounding Salt Lake City.

Then, one Sunday morning at 6:30, my pager went off. "Lord Jesus!" I exclaimed to my wife. "They have a heart for me!" I was right: IMC did have a transplantable heart ready, or would, as soon as it was harvested from the donor. I went to church that morning and shared my excitement with my friends, and I got to the hospital before noon. But it was hurry-up-and-wait, because the heart is the last organ to be harvested from a body. (Most heart transplant surgeries are performed in the middle of the night.) After I had been prepped for the surgery, I was left alone in the hallway outside the surgery room, where I had about twelve hours to pray and reflect on what was about to happen. I felt some doubt about the surgery, because the LVAD installation had been traumatic, but I felt spiritually cared for and supported, both by God and by my support system of family and friends. Everybody knew everybody, and I knew I wasn't there alone.

I awoke at noon the next day, after a night of surgery, and everything was new. Wired from the prednisone[xxv] I'd been given, I didn't sleep for two days. I also had blood clots in both arms. But these were minor problems at this point. I wasn't exactly resurrected, but it was like night and day difference. I hadn't felt that way in probably eleven years.

I had to stay in Salt Lake City for recovery for another eleven months.[xxvi] I finally came home to Albuquerque in October 2013.

My life now is still punctuated by trips to Salt Lake City for checkups, and it is regulated by the handful of drugs I take to keep my body and my new heart agreeable with each other. But I'm not just a patient any more: I'm active with a campus Christian club at the University of New Mexico, and I'm riding my bike.

More than anything, I am thankful for my relationships, beginning with my wife. When we said these vows when we got married, we had no idea what we were saying — "I take thee in health and in health, for better or for better." My poor wife, I don't think she ever dreamed of being a caregiver. Thinking of her stoicism makes me cry. There are a lot of people where the spouse gets ill, and they just leave… I just feel so blessed that she would stay and help me. I also recall friends from New Heart that sent me letters in the hospital, some of whom have themselves died. It was just amazing, the support. In contrast, I consider my older brother, who died of heart failure only last year. Unlike me, my brother had lived alone. He'd had a chance to get an LVAD, on the condition that he quit smoking,[xxvii] but he hadn't been able to quit on his own.

My main advice for fellow sufferers is to be with others — others who will pray with you and support you, others who are a step ahead of you in rehabilitation.

My second piece of advice is to reconsider the meaning of suffering. Suffering gives you different perspectives. Some people can become hardened and bitter, but the Lord himself suffered his whole life. There are a lot of different aspects of life that we need to really appreciate it.

3.   The (Meta)Astrophysicist

Editors' introduction

As an astrophysicist at the New Mexico Institute of Mining and Technology, Dr. David Westpfahl spends his professional life understanding numbers. Naturally, then, when he underwent heart surgery in 2007, he used his skills in quantitative analysis to help himself prepare for his ordeal, and to measure his rehabilitation afterward. But his experience shows that there are forces in the realm of cardiac intervention and rehabilitation that transcend the rationality of numbers.

Dave's story

The hardest part about getting heart surgery was preparing for my own death. I had life insurance, and that's an indication that I had thought something about it. But to make real plans — to write down, "I want to be cremated, I want to be buried in the family plot in Dunmore, Pennsylvania" — that is irreversible. I knew from my professional field, astrophysics, that there are irreversible events or processes. But I also knew that mathematical probabilities could be trusted if you applied your analytical mind to them.

Probability was the cause of my heart problem in the first place. My uncles on my mom's side had all suffered from unusual aortic valves: they were bicuspid rather than tricuspid.[xxviii] I'd inherited that trait, but I'd always been fit. When I was 52, I went on a safari, and the tour guide told me I was a strong walker. But a year later, I got the distinct feeling that I was losing strength, slowing down with age. In my annual physical, my primary doctor told me the sound of my heart had changed. It didn't even occur to me to ask why at first — I'd been told there were funny sounds coming from my heart my whole life.[xxix] I think my doctor knew there was something wrong, though, because he referred me to a cardiologist. It turned out that my aortic valve was not only bicuspid, but it had also become calcified; it was .7 cm2 rather than the normal 4 cm2. I was going to need valve replacement. It had been a concern of mine for a long time, so in some ways it was not a surprise.

The surgeon told me there was a 2% chance I'd die during surgery and another 2% chance I'd die during recovery. I had to apply my analytical skill and convince myself that this task had to be accomplished. If my surgeon was a baseball player, he'd be batting .960. Was that good enough? My mathematical mind told me it was; my professional training told me that if you analyze something with mathematics and you come to a conclusion, you may not like the conclusion, but it may be undeniable. Okay, I had to prepare for my own death. I didn't like that conclusion, but it was the right answer.

I still spent a couple of weeks dragging my feet. Ultimately, what motivated me was providing for my wife, who is disabled by MS and Parkinson's. So my heart convinced my head to act.

As I waited out the six months between my diagnosis and my surgery, one thing I didn't do was pray. I'd been raised Episcopalian, but the pivotal religious moment of my life had been when I'd been kicked out of Sunday School at age 4 for refusing to make a coloring-book Jesus look Aryan. Two nights before my surgery, though, I had a dream that defied rational explanation.

In the dream, I was surrounded by several older people. A woman of mixed Spanish and Native American heritage spoke to me: "You're going to do very well."

"Are you God?" I asked.

She answered, "No, we're God's servants, and we have more work for you. We can't tell you what the outcome is going to be, but you're going to do very well."

Did I make that up? Did some other agent speak to me? Was it just a dream? I have no way to answer these questions. But I did feel comforted by the dream; and to this day, I feel as though I have been assigned work.

I also had an uncanny experience during my surgery: the anesthesiologist had put me completely under, but I distinctly remember hearing a doctor put three wires in my sternum and talk about using adhesive to glue me back together. After the surgery, I told the doc about my memory, and he turned ashen. He left the room and came back with a psychiatrist.

The shrink said, "What do you make of that?"

I told him, "Well, I knew I'd made it. I knew I'd survive. It gave me great confidence that I was going to wake up."

Ultimately, heart surgery gave me some lessons about consciousness, but the lesson I learned from recovering from heart surgery was patience. I spent six days in the hospital and another week at home. It was slow, and I felt pain whenever I sneezed. I realized that my recovery rate was like the Gibbs energy in thermal physics[xxx]: it had a finite potential. I couldn't control the rate of my healing unless I was patient. If I was patient, it could go as fast as it could go; if I was impatient, I would slow it down.

Fortunately, I had New Heart's staff to help me achieve my best potential recovery rate. The people I met here were pulling for my success; it was the whole spirit of the place. Everyone was friendly and welcoming, and the staff did everything they could not to make this feel like another medical appointment. They kept an eye on me, made sure I didn't push too hard — the initial daily walking goal they gave me was eight minutes on the treadmill at two miles per hour with 13 minutes of additional exercise on other machines.

One day, about two months into rehab, I told myself I was going to do an hour on the treadmill. I walked 3.6 miles. That's when I knew I was back.

At that point, I set my own goal: one million steps in 80 days. To reach this goal, I had two daily walking sessions. During the day, I would spend one hour walking continuously at four miles per hour. After dinner, I would take another two-mile walk. I wound up reaching my 1,000,000th step on day 73.

Once I met that goal, I saw how I could stretch it. I realized that 5 x 73 = 365, so I could realistically walk 5 million steps in a year. I gradually increased my walking goals over the next two years, working up to 25,000 steps per day, or 9,000,000 steps per year, about 4500 miles. I eventually set the goal of walking 25,000 miles in six years — 25,000 miles because that is the equatorial circumference of the Earth.

I made sure I was at New Heart when I hit my goal. It was on March 2, 2015, in the afternoon. There were about a dozen people working out at New Heart. I got on a treadmill to complete the goal, which took about 15 minutes. Dr. Lueker made an announcement to everyone when I took the 50,000,000th step.

I'm still motivated by numbers: I walk 25,000 steps every day, and I log all my miles with a pedometer. In the last six years, I've walked 25,800 miles — more than the circumference of the Earth. As a quantitative analyst, I know this is really about bringing my professional skills to bear on my exercise. However, as a member of the New Heart board, I'm mainly motivated to be an example for new patients. When I was an early patient, I would look at people ahead of me and tell myself, "In two months, I could be doing that." Now I'm compelled to be the best teacher I can be. Some new patients are like students of mine who won't do their homework, and like my students, I tell them that the doing is the most important part. The number of steps is not terribly important, the speed is not terribly important; it's the doing, every day, that's important.

4.   The Worldly Priest

Editors' introduction

The first thing one notices about Father Francis Dorff is his eyes: shining with interest and engagement, these are the eyes of an 81-year old who is in love with the world and the connections that bind it. Reflecting on his 20-year struggle with heart disease, the priest/theologian/philosopher spends more time talking about the nurses and doctors he's met than he spends talking about himself.

Francis's story

My first instance of heart disease occurred over twenty years ago, when I filled in for a mentor with heart disease. I was studying with depth psychologist Dr. Ira Progoff at a retreat center in California, when he suffered a heart attack and was rushed to the hospital. I was tapped to run the class. Fearing that the other students would be displeased about the substitution, I spent the night before my first lesson tossing and turning. But I was feeling more than stress: I felt pain in my chest while breathing. I didn't think of heart trouble, though — it felt to me like a case of pleurisy.[xxxi]

Although I thought my trouble might be with my stomach, I felt that my vital signs were off — and apparently they were. The next day, I asked the staff nurse at the retreat center if she could take my pulse, but she couldn't find it, and she just walked away. Confused, but accepting the nurse's authority, I returned to my own therapy center in New

Mexico's Jemez Mountains. There, I asked a visiting Tai Chi master to take my pulse. After holding his hand above my wrist for a few seconds, his eyes widened with alarm, and he told me to go to intensive care immediately.

I spent the next ten days in intensive care at Presbyterian Hospital, losing energy because my heart was fibrillating.[xxxii] I had a hard time accepting my illness: for eight of those ten days, I was arguing with God, telling Him, "My work's not finished." Answers from God aren't uncommon for me, but it usually takes fifteen years or so! However, this one came through when I was still in the hospital: "Francis, you have it all wrong... I don't take you when your work's finished; when I take you, then your work's finished."

During this first hospital stay, I found that my inquisitive nature prompted different reactions from different doctors. The first doctor assigned to me was clearly in a hurry and would try to enter and exit my room quickly. When I stopped him once to ask about my condition, the impatient doctor retorted, "I know what kind of guy you are. You're the kind who asks questions." Taken aback, I answered, "I'm a philosopher — I ask questions for a living." I started looking for another doctor, someone who would communicate fully with me. One day, I overheard Dr. Catherine Blake briefing nurses in the room next door. Appreciating the clarity with which she spoke, I approached her to take over as my doctor. I'm glad I did.

When I was discharged from Presbyterian, I went straight into rehabilitation at New Heart. I recognized immediately that it was a sacred place, more like a temple than a medical center. It wasn't religious, it wasn't ritualistic; it just had an integrity of purpose. The building was alive with people getting well, being guided by all of these healers. And the patients were helping one another, too.

After three months of rehabilitation, I returned to my abbey, the Norbertine Community of Santa María de la Vid. I resumed my daily walks in the desert, supplemented with sessions on a stationary bike.

I would have happily put my heart troubles behind me if they hadn't returned sixteen years later.

Again, my stomach spoke for my heart. Four years ago, I came down with what felt like a terrible case of acid reflux. I saw Dr. Blake about it, and she sent me to the Heart Hospital right away. Indeed, I had blockages in my right coronary artery, my left leg, and my carotid arteries. I underwent angioplasty[xxxiii] to flush out my blocked arteries.

You might have thought that I would be angry or depressed about returning to the hospital for a second cardiac intervention; actually, I became sort of euphoric. There's a peacefulness in it. Some patients are really arrogant — it's their chance to play king — but I loved to sit and talk with the nurses and learn about their lives. I have such an admiration for them — it's such a dedicated life. The hospital is a place of suffering, but it's full of peaceful people who have dedicated their lives to healing. I was also fascinated by watching my own heart on a monitor when they would take ultrasounds.

After several days in the heart hospital, I returned to New Heart for rehabilitation. Once again, I found it restorative on many levels. To see the older people working at their own rates, and all supportive of one another — that was very, very supportive for me. New Heart is a good extension of the operating room. And it's a work of dedication, so it's a labor of love, and you can feel that.

Since then, my circulatory system has been relatively stable, though I still have some minor blockages and calcifications.[xxxiv] I still have to have open heart surgery.

What meaning do I make of my struggle? It really calls me to a deeper personal relationship with the body, and with the wisdom of the body. In the meditative writing that I practice, any aspect of my life can be animated by contemplative dialogue. I become quiet and present to the body, and I can speak with it about its present situation, or about my anxieties or whatever, and it's amazing: it becomes like a spiritual director to me. So I honor the body by marking out its basic steppingstones — what it has lived through. And then all kinds of leads will come from there, from the energies that are in that dialogue, that relationship, and where these energies want to go.

Ultimately, I see suffering to be coextensive with the spiritual church. I'm a student of Teresa of Ávila, the 16th-century Spanish saint. Saint Teresa writes about the "interior castle," or the soul's dwelling place as I like to call it — a magnificent interior mansion composed of seven rooms through which we experience God's presence more and more intimately. Every step along the way is carrying a dark night — it has a suffering component of the body, mind, or soul. In other words, life is a mystery that can only be accessed by suffering.

So my advice to a fellow heart disease sufferer is to let your body be your guide by being compassionately attentive to it. That sets up a whole new spiritual possibility.

5.   The Anxious Convalescent

Editors' introduction

In the processes of intervention and rehabilitation, most heart attack survivors are given a clear reason for their heart disease, and consequently, a clear path to recovery. This wasn't the case with "Helen," who had no family history of heart disease and no obvious causes for her own. This ambiguity has made her anxious about which elements of her lifestyle to improve. As you'll see, though, that hasn't stopped her from trying.

Helen's story

A month before my heart attack, I started getting this feeling like something was sitting on my chest. When it would come on, it made my arms tired, and I could feel weird tingling sensations going down my arms as if they were going to sleep. I thought it was my job — I'd recently started working at a new company, and it was turning out to be a very stressful environment. Unfortunately, I seem to attract stressful jobs. Anyway, I didn't really think anything was wrong with me but I thought to be on the safe side, I should check with my primary care provider. I made an appointment with him, and he ran an EKG. My EKG results and my blood pressure were satisfactory, and when I left his office, he told me he hoped that this would be the last time we discussed this. That comment continues to haunt me.

Several weeks later, I got up at 5:30 and jogged for thirty minutes on the treadmill. When I got in the shower, I felt pains going across my back and down my arms. Then I felt short of breath and started to sweat. I decided to wash off and soon realized that I didn't have the energy to push the pump on the soap dispenser. At that point, I knew I'd better get some help.

I called for my husband, and thankfully, he was still in the bedroom and heard me. He helped me out of the shower, and we called Ask-a-Nurse. The nurse asked a number of questions, the majority of which got "yes" answers, and informed us that we should call 911. We spent a half hour on the phone establishing our address and other miscellaneous information with 911. Finally, 911 concluded that we should either head to an emergency room, or they would dispatch an ambulance. Mainly because we didn't want to leave our 11-year old son at home alone, we asked them to send an ambulance.

Fortunately, the EMTs arrived quickly, recognized a cardiac event in my symptoms, and got me to the Heart Hospital of New Mexico very quickly. I was later informed that this decision was extremely helpful in getting me the care I needed quickly and likely prevented damage to my heart. The first doctor I met at the Heart Hospital told me, "You're having a heart attack. But the good news is that you're here early in the morning, all our doctors are here, and all of the operating rooms are available." Within 15 minutes, I was getting an angioplasty. A stent was inserted into my LAD artery, which was 100% clogged.

The hardest part of being in the hospital that first time was the visitors. My parents showed up first because my son had called them. Then a bunch of coworkers came to see me, including the president of my new company. I'd come to the hospital right out of the shower, so my hair was flat and I had no makeup on; it was pretty embarrassing. I do have to mention though that the people at the Heart Hospital were wonderful.

Three days later, back at home, I started feeling the same symptoms again — pain in my back and arms, shortness of breath, weakness. I went right back to the Heart Hospital, and they discovered that I had a blood clot in the new stent. They performed a second angioplasty, removed the blood clot and slightly extended the stent.

I was very paranoid for the first four to six months after my second angioplasty. I lost around ten pounds because I was afraid to eat anything. I didn't want to go anywhere outside of Albuquerque, because I wanted to be near the Heart Hospital in case anything happened. One evening, about a month after the heart attack, I felt my blood pressure getting too high, so I took a nitroglycerin pill.[xxxv] The nitroglycerin ended up lowering my blood pressure so much that we ended up calling an ambulance, and I went back to the Heart Hospital. Luckily, the doctors found that my heart was not in distress, and I learned a lesson about the effects of nitroglycerin.

The worst part of the whole experience was that I had this new health concern with no logical explanation for it. Both of my parents have high blood pressure, but nobody in my family has suffered a heart attack. I had very minor increased cholesterol, but I rarely ate anything fried; I exercised regularly; I didn't smoke. I kept asking why I had the heart attack, and I never got a solid answer. That's the part that really kind of still bothers me.

The ambiguity of my heart condition made me ambivalent about rehabilitation at first. The people at the Heart Hospital told me about New Heart, and that the statistics were good for people that went there and did what they needed to do. But I had already been pretty fit. If my problem had been more pronounced, and I could stop whatever that problem was to recuperate, I probably would have been less likely to start cardiac rehab. However, since there was no obvious outlying cause for my heart attack, I thought, "Well, the least I could do is not eat less salt and try New Heart."

When I started rehabilitation at New Heart, it was freaky at first to be hooked up to the heart monitors while I was on the cardio machines, especially when the monitoring tech[xxxvi] told me to slow down. It was also a bit unsettling to be back on a treadmill, since my heart attack had happened right after I had been on a treadmill. (I take very quick showers nowadays for the same reason.) I truly enjoyed my single one-on-one meeting with New Heart's dietician, though. My insurance would only pay for one meeting, but I took notes and have tried to incorporate more healthy foods, and healthy cooking, into my diet. New Heart also had a stress class, which was very helpful as well because it allowed me to visit with other people who had similar experiences and feelings, and it was very reassuring to hear their concerns and know that I wasn't alone.

Ultimately, I kept returning to New Heart to do my workouts because I knew they knew my story, and if anything went wrong, they would know what to do to help me. It's actually kind of freaky now to exercise without the monitors!

After about a year of being at New Heart, I saw tangible results from my cardiologist that the rehab was working. He was pleased with the frequency of my visits, and the blood pressure records on my chart showed that the exercise was indeed making a difference. My paranoia decreased a lot at that point. I have noticed that I stay healthier, from a cold and flu standpoint, when I exercise regularly. New Heart has also taught me some great stress-management exercises.

But my fears about my heart haven't entirely disappeared. My doctor sometimes makes me feel stupid for worrying, but I just do. It's maddening... I don't know what to do to keep a heart attack from happening again. I've reduced salt in my diet, and I go to New Heart to exercise. I'm on Crestor[xxxvii] as of very recently because my cholesterol is still a little high. Those are about the only changes I've made.

I think I need to be a little more balanced in terms of work and peace. I have recently found another job, which is less stressful. The hard part is finding the time to go to New Heart to exercise. My new employer is across town, so if it's after 5:30, I just can't make it, because I don't get to New Heart until 6, and then I don't get home until 7:30, and my 13-year old needs supervision between those hours. I hope to start doing yoga soon.

My advice to others is to absolutely give cardiac rehab at try, because it's reassuring that people know what's going on with you and can support you. They don't care whether you look like an idiot on the treadmill, whether you're sweating and your makeup's running. You don't have to look perfect. It's a caring, family kind of environment.

6. The Iron Horse

Editors' introduction

Durand Smith's story of running the Iron Horse Bicycle Classic has been one of Dr. Lueker's favorite anecdotes for years — not only because it shows successful recovery from heart disease, but because the manner of Durand's success was so exciting. To go from a hospital bed to a 55-mile bike race in just a few months is a phenomenal feat of human strength and willpower, as well as a testament to the impact of cardiac rehabilitation.

Durand's story

I've always been a cyclist, but it took a heart attack and a triple bypass to make me a truly strong rider.

A decade ago, when I was in my late fifties, I wasn't riding much. My work as a manager in the aerospace industry made me put in long hours. I noticed that I wasn't feeling myself — tired, run-down — so I went to my physician. But he couldn't find anything wrong with me. I kept riding on the weekends, but I felt limited.

My heart attack came on a Saturday when I was home alone. I was out feeding my wife's pet chicken, and all of a sudden I felt very light-headed. I lay down on a patch of grass and passed out. My doctor told me later that my heart stopped when I was out, so it's miraculous that I even woke up. When I did wake up, I didn't know the problem was my heart; I was more alarmed that I'd wet my pants while I was unconscious. I hobbled into the house and called one of my daughters, who called 911 (it didn't occur to me to do that). The EMTs took me right to the heart hospital, and my heart stopped again when I was talking to a doctor there.

The cardiologists' first intervention was putting in a stent. But they knew afterward that the stent didn't do it, because the blockage was too extensive. So they decided to do a bypass surgery the next day. It wound up being a triple bypass.[xxxviii]

I remember being put on the operating table: it felt like a cold slab as one of the doctors was about to administer the anesthetic. My next moment of consciousness was in the hospital bed. It's an experience, with all of the tubes and things sticking out of you.

I was impatient to get out of the hospital after my surgery, so I was trying to do whatever I could to get better. I was encouraged to get up for the bathroom and walk. Within two days I was walking the halls. My surgery was on a Sunday, and I was home by the next Friday.

I was referred to New Heart by the heart hospital, and I was anxious to be able to get started in rehabilitation. But I was very weak. In the introductory tour of New Heart, I was probably the weakest one there — I had to sit down a lot.

Although I was weak at first, I wanted to be pushing myself a little bit harder than what I was encouraged to do. I've always believed in the axiom, No pain, no gain. But I wasn't sweating at all as I was working out, so I didn't think I was doing very much to help myself. In retrospect, I can see that Dr. Lueker and the New Heart staff knew the right way to heal; but at the time, I felt like I was being held back.

Several months into rehab, I started riding my bike again. I felt I had to do something where I could push the envelope out far enough so that any other activity that I would normally do would not cause me any concern about my physical abilities. So I set a steep goal: to ride the Iron Horse Bicycle Classic — a 55-mile race through the Colorado mountains from Durango to Silverton, climbing over two 10,000-foot peaks. My son-in-law, who manages a bike store, pledged to ride the race with me, and we trained together. I worried in the beginning about having another attack, but I just kept pushing myself. I knew I was on my way when we rode from Albuquerque to the top of the Sandia Mountains.

I completed the Iron Horse only 11 months after my heart attack. I was not the fastest — I was trying to get my son-in-law to take off and ride with the other people that were closer to his abilities — but he stuck with me the whole way. By the time I got to the finish line, they were taking down the race course. But my wife and all three of my daughters were there to see me finish. That was a great day.

I went back to work after taking a couple of months off. I knew that I had to make some lifestyle changes and I gave up my job as a manager of over a hundred engineers to become an individual contributor once more. I also made exercise part of my work day. As I interviewed for new assignments, I made it clear that my normal routine would be coming in early, eating lunch at my desk, and leaving at 3 pm to work out at New Heart. I was fortunate that everyone accepted this. In fact, people often reminded me when it was 3 o'clock.

I retired a year ago, and I have been spending summers in Maine and winters in New Mexico. The biggest challenge I have now is keeping up with the exercise. The primary issue is having a routine to follow and exercising regularly. I still ride, and I am fortunate that in summers I can take walks along an ocean path and ride a 20-mile loop in one of the most beautiful places on earth, Acadia National Park.

7.   The Mountaineer

Editors' introduction

Rudy's story is a triumph of victory over life events and heart disease. His illness produced profound weakness, but he has recovered dramatically and continues to work, literally climbing mountains and figuratively exploring avenues of his profession. His story is a perfect illustration of the positive feedback loop of effort and energy.

Rudy's story

I'm mister macho, from way back. I served 20 years in the Air Force, worked 22 years at Sandia National Laboratories (NM), and in 2003 started a civil engineering consulting company. I've always worked hard and played hard. Every summer for the last 31+ years, my buddies and I have gone backpacking in the mountains. I carry a 40-pound pack for five or six days. So nine years back, when I suddenly couldn't make the walk to my mailbox, I had no idea what was going on. I'd never had heart problems; I never thought this would happen to me.

I was in my late 60s in March of 2007. I'd spent the last three years going through a divorce. Emotionally, I was expecting some kind of hangover from that, but I sure didn't expect any physical reactions. Then my stomach started giving me trouble: my GI system went out of whack, my stomach was hurting, and I couldn't eat as much as usual. (My mother and father came from central Italy, so they certainly taught me how I to throw down some serious pasta and bread.) Then one day, out of the blue, I was unable to walk to my mailbox. I figured I had a little bug and took the day off. But a couple days later, I couldn't walk from my bathroom to my sofa.

I called my lady-friend at the time (now my second wife), and told her I couldn't get up. She told me to call an ambulance. I didn't want to (mister macho, remember), but she came over and insisted. When the EMTs showed up and took my blood pressure, they said it was 250. That made me jump up from the sofa — I suddenly remembered that my dad had died of a heart attack when he was sweeping snow from the driveway at 87 — and the EMTs made me lie down again on their stretcher. I had to face the fact that I was seriously ill. Good thing I'd been in a 12-step program at that time for over 20 years, which gave me the ability to face reality and deal with any predicament head-on.

I spent three days in the hospital getting tests. I had so much trust in all the doctors, even though I was mad at them because they couldn't agree on what was wrong. On the fourth day, four doctors came into my room and told me their theories. A couple of them thought I might have blockages in my guts, since I was mostly feeling pain there. Dr. Harvey White, the cardiologist attending me, thought there might be a blockage under my heart, which they couldn't see with the tests they'd been running. He wanted to do an angioplasty. I agreed to that the next day; when they did it, they showed me that my LAD[xxxix] had 95% blockage. I could see it on the monitor even though I was sedated. They put a stent in to clear out the blockage.

I went home that Saturday, but I still wasn't feeling completely well: I still had gut pains. So I went back to the hospital on the following Tuesday. A rheumatologist attending to me thought I had polymyalgia rheumatica.[xl] But I had started feeling terrible pain and pressure in my chest, in addition to the gut pains. I also began gasping for air. They rushed me to surgery and went straight into my LAD again, and found that it had kinked right above the first stent.[xli] So a second cardiologist put another stent (in tandem) above the first one. They also gave me a big shot of prednisone, which made my bowels finally start moving. After that was over, I felt like a new man.

When I got home, I got a call from the wife of one of my skiing buddies, who worked at New Heart. She suggested their cardiac rehabilitation program to me, and I wanted to try it right away, because it would put me on a routine so I could continue with my backpacking plans that July (within only 4 months).

My rehabilitation was hard and fast. I started going to New Heart three times a week; I wanted to get well so badly that I wasn't going to play any games. I'm the kind of guy that, once I commit, I commit. Especially if I see a purpose. The New Heart staff made me slow down on the treadmill once or twice because I was going too fast. I trusted their advice, but I wasn't afraid of having another heart problem at that point. Dr. White had told me my heart was good, and I mainly needed to work on my cholesterol. I enrolled in the Prevent Heart Disease (PHD) Program.[xlii] I got very good at self-monitoring: I could feel when I pushed past 135 bpm.

After about a month, I got off the monitors. Two or three months out, I got a stress test. The testers told me I was stronger than a lot of younger guys. They checked me out for backpacking, under the condition that I would wear a heart monitor and not go over 130 bpm.

Working out at New Heart was part of why I recovered so quickly, but the other important element was prayer. My new wife is an All-Faiths Minister, and we prayed together often. I felt still young — under 70 — and I had a second life, which I was not about to waste.

I went backpacking in July, as planned. My five buddies kept a close eye on me, and I kept a close eye on that heart monitor. It was an incredible trip — 6 days hiking over 12,000 feet — and I loved it because I deserved it: I had followed instructions, I didn't pooh-pooh it, and I'd prayed a lot.

I'm 78 now, so I'm slowing down a bit. I've substituted my more dangerous sports — whitewater rafting and downhill skiing — for ones where I'm on firm ground — like cross-country skiing and hiking. I'm still backpacking, but I'm wiser about it: I leave my heavier gear at a campsite and go day-hiking more. I can push myself a little bit, because I'm not wearing myself out, I'm not killing myself; I'm actually giving myself life. I feel balanced and stable, like I have a solid foundation.

My family comments on my excellent health all the time. My wife says my reflexes are phenomenal, and my kids and grandchildren ask me where I get all my energy. That always gives me a boost.

When I meditate, sometimes I ask God, "What more do I need to do?" The response I get is, "Keep going. You can do it — get out there and do it. You've got the energy. I've given you the body and I've given you the brains. Get out there and do it!"

My father taught me about giving your gifts back to others — "If you get it, pass it on." I'm grateful because I can still serve people. Recently, I helped my sister recover from a couple of hip surgeries. She's just a year older than me, but she was laid up. She could only listen to me tell her what it was like to walking around the golf course by her house. I almost felt guilty that I could do it and she couldn't. I'm also working with a think tank on evaluating infrastructure deterioration and enhanced security, and on designing for longer-lasting structures and systems (more facility sustainability). What a reward, to be at my age, and still be able to contribute.

My advice: perseverance. Meditation. Commitment. It all comes with hard work, but the reward is a higher quality of life and enhanced service to others.

About the Authors

Richard D. Lueker, M.D., F.A.C.C., F.A.C.P.

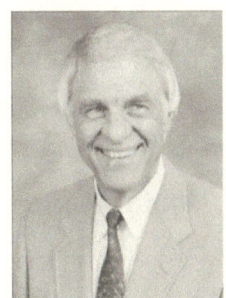

Richard D. Lueker has been a member of the medical community in Albuquerque since he joined the faculty of the University of New Mexico School of Medicine. He graduated from the University of Colorado School of Medicine, completed two years of Internal Medicine Residency at the University of Minnesota prior to spending two years in Thailand serving as a fraternal worker at the Bangkok Christian Hospital. He retuned to the University of Colorado School of Medicine, where he completed his medical residency, serving as Chief Medical Resident for one year. He then completed two years in cardiology fellowship training at Colorado under the direction of S. Gilbert Bount.

During that time, he was actively engaged in cardiovascular research trials resulting in presentations and national meetings. After completing a year in transplantation research, he was recruited to join the University of New Mexico School of Medicine, where he was an Assistant Professor in the Cardiology Division.

With Dr. Ralph Williams, he visited the Rheumatic Fever Hospital in Cairo, Egypt, studying altered lymphocyte reactivity in such patients.

In 1975, with two University of New Mexico colleagues, Professors Atterbom and Gustafson, Lueker developed the New Heart Cardiac Rehabilitation and Prevention Program, a 501c3 nonprofit entity. In conjunction with Presbyterian Hospital of Albuquerque, the New Heart Healthplex was constructed. In 2005, a multimillion dollar gift from Blake Chanslor made possible the construction of a new freestanding center near downtown Albuquerque. Since that time, the New Heart program has served thousands of patients in cardiac rehabilitation and prevention programs.

Christopher J. Ritter, Ph.D.

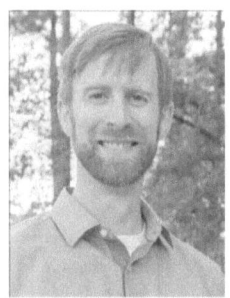

Christopher J. Ritter has taught at the college level since 2002 in literature, rhetoric and composition, and digital humanities. He earned his doctorate from Washington State University in 2010, under the guidance of Victor Villanueva, Patricia Freitag Ericsson, and Jason Farman. His doctoral research concentrated on digital rhetoric, particularly in digital games. He has completed graduate coursework in the analysis, composition, and pedagogy of contemporary and digital rhetoric, technical communication, and literature.

From 2010 to 2013, he held a Marion L. Brittain Postdoctoral Fellowship at the Georgia Institute of Technology, in which he ran a client-based technical communication course that provided communication consulting for local nonprofits, small businesses, and startups. In 2013-14, he co-taught a pilot version of technical communication that was integrated with the School of Computer Science's capstone design projects course, in which student teams planned, composed, and delivered client-based and entrepreneurial applications over two semesters. Since 2014, he has been an Assistant Professor in the English Department at Clayton State University.

Ritter has published individually and collaboratively on his teaching; presented at local, regional, national, and international conferences; led workshops on pedagogy and digital technologies; guest-lectured on teaching, digital rhetoric, and literature; and given interviews on studying and teaching games. His writing focuses on teaching, rhetoric, art, history, and his family.

Notes

i **145/110:** Normal blood pressure is in the range of 120 mm over 80 mm. The first number, 120 mm, is the result of the heart's pumping action — the pressure produced by forcing blood out of the heart. The second, or lower number, is the diastolic pressure which is the effect of the arteries' shape. If the artery constricts, narrows, the diastolic pressure goes up. If the artery is relaxed, the diastolic pressure should be 80 mm or even lower. If the diastolic pressure is higher, over time, this produces more stress on the heart muscle, the left ventricle, which is the pump that pushes blood through the body's circulatory system. Additionally, elevated pressure is also associated with the development of blockages within the coronary arteries that furnish blood to the heart muscle.

ii **a statin:** "Statins are drugs that can lower your cholesterol. They work by blocking a substance your body needs to make cholesterol. Statins may also help your body reabsorb cholesterol that has built up in plaques on your artery walls, preventing further blockage in your blood vessels and heart attacks. Statins include medications such as atorvastatin (Lipitor), fluvastatin (Lescol), lovastatin (Altoprev), pitavastatin (Livalo), pravastatin (Pravachol), rosuvastatin (Crestor) and simvastatin (Zocor). Lower-cost generic versions of many statin medications are available." Source: http://www.mayoclinic.org/statins/art-20045772

iii **a big stent in my main coronary artery:** In an angioplasty, the goal of the cardiologist is to open the artery that is blocked, and thus to restore blood flow to the tissue that it supplies. If the artery remains closed, the tissue it supplies may die, which may cause significant complications. Thus, opening of the artery, if possible, is essential.

A small thin wire is passed though the artery, through the blockage. Riding on the wire is a small balloon, which is not inflated. When the balloon is adjacent to (within) the blockage, the balloon is then inflated, and the blockage may be reduced and pushed back. This permits blood to flow through the vessel to the needy tissue. Then it is possible to place a small wire mesh, called a *stent*, into the area where the block occurred to prevent the re-closure collapse of the artery again. The collapsed stent is moved into position by the cardiologist. When it reaches the area where the blockage was present, the stent is expanded, supporting and expanding the wall of the artery, preventing it from closing again. The balloon is then deflated and removed, and the stent remains in place within the artery wall.

iv **Ischemia:** This means "lack of oxygen," inadequate amount of oxygen to the tissue which was to be supplied by the artery. If the artery is narrowed briefly, as a result of spasm, the tissue supplied will not die. If the closure is more prolonged, the tissue supplied by the artery may die. In the heart this may result in a myocardial infarction (a heart attack). If the affected artery is in the brain, the result would be a stroke.

v **scared me:** After experiencing a heart attack, someone usually feels a significant amount of concern, worry, anxiety or even fear about another heart attack. It is not unusual that the person has increased sensitivity to "feelings" in the body and chest. Gradually, daily, weekly, monthly, as a person experiences a faster heart rate while feeling strong and wonderful, the person realizes that they are much healthier than they were before. As time goes on with ever-increasing activity and increasing heart rate, the person recognizes, "I am ok…. I am not hurting myself." Due to the increase in physical activity, hormones within the body increase to assist in greater self-confidence and less fear, assisting in more happiness and peace. Thus, the hypersensitivity, anxiety, and fear are gradually replaced by the awareness that "I am better than I have ever been. I could never have done this before my heart attack. I am stronger than I have been in years."

vi **don't be scared:** A heart attack can be an opportunity to learn and respect the feelings of the body. Someone who undergoes cardiac rehabilitation learns what "risk" factors led to their problem, what led to their heart event. They study these issues, and they attack them. As time goes on, they become more and more aware of their physical and emotional progress. They get to know their body more intimately than ever before. Fear and anxiety are replaced by greater and greater self-confidence. This builds as they realize that their strength and energy are better than they've been in years, better than people five or ten years younger than they are. Individuals feel joy and confidence that they have made such progress. Thus, many times those who were victims now begin to see themselves as victors.

vii **heart murmur:** "Heart murmurs are sounds during your heartbeat cycle – such as whooshing or swishing – made by turbulent blood in or near your heart. These sounds can be heard with a stethoscope. A normal heartbeat makes two

sounds like "lubb-dupp" (sometimes described as "lub-DUP"), which are the sounds of your heart valves closing."
Source: http://www.mayoclinic.org/diseases-conditions/heart-murmurs/basics/definition/con-20028706

viii **prolapsed mitral valve:** "Mitral valve prolapse (MVP) occurs when the valve between your heart's left upper chamber (left atrium) and the left lower chamber (left ventricle) doesn't close properly. During mitral valve prolapse, the leaflets of the mitral valve bulge (prolapse) upward or back into the left atrium as the heart contracts. Mitral valve prolapse sometimes leads to blood leaking backward into the left atrium, a condition called mitral valve regurgitation."
Source: http://www.mayoclinic.org/diseases-conditions/mitral-valve-prolapse/basics/definition/con-20024748

ix **severe mitral valve regurgitation with cardiomyopathy**: Gregg's heart function had been reduced by a third, and its ejection fraction was at 40%.

x **mitral valve repair with a Delran ring:** "In mitral valve repair, a doctor removes the portion of the mitral valve that doesn't close properly. ... Then a doctor sutures together the edges and cinches the circumference of the valve with an annuloplasty band to support the valve." Source: http://www.mayoclinic.org/diseases-conditions/mitral-valve-disease/multimedia/mitral-valve-repair/img-20123830

xi **arrhythmia:** "Heart rhythm problems (heart arrhythmias) occur when the electrical impulses that coordinate your heartbeats don't work properly, causing your heart to beat too fast, too slow or irregularly. Heart arrhythmias (uh-RITH-meuhs) may feel like a fluttering or racing heart and may be harmless. However, some heart arrhythmias may cause bothersome – sometimes even life-threatening – signs and symptoms." Source: http://www.mayoclinic.org/diseases-conditions/heart-arrhythmia/basics/definition/con-20027707

xii **ventricular tachycardia:** "Ventricular tachycardia is a heart rhythm disorder (arrhythmia) caused by abnormal electrical signals in the lower chambers of the heart (ventricles). Your heart rate is regulated by electrical signals sent across heart tissues. A healthy heart normally beats about 60 to 100 times a minute when at rest and is defined by signals that originate in the upper chambers of the heart (atria). In ventricular tachycardia (V-tach or VT), abnormal electrical signals in the ventricles cause the heart to beat faster than normal, usually 100 or more beats a minute, out of sync with the upper chambers." Source: https://www.mayoclinic.org/diseases-conditions/ventricular-tachycardia/symptoms-causes/syc-20355138

xiii **Implanted Cardio Defibrillator (ICD):** "Implantable cardioverter-defibrillators work by detecting and stopping abnormal heartbeats (arrhythmias). An implantable cardioverter-defibrillator continuously monitors your heartbeat and delivers extra beats or electrical shocks to restore a normal heart rhythm when necessary." Source: http://www.mayoclinic.org/tests-procedures/implantable-cardioverter-defibrillator/basics/definition/prc-20015079

xiv **a dent that wouldn't go away:** These symptoms occur because blood accumulates in the lungs, which causes shortness of breath. Poor heart muscle function causes reduced return of blood flow back to the heart, thus resulting in "pooling" of the blood and swelling of the legs.

xv **congestive heart failure:** "Heart failure, sometimes known as congestive heart failure, occurs when your heart muscle doesn't pump blood as well as it should. Certain conditions, such as narrowed arteries in your heart (coronary artery disease) or high blood pressure, gradually leave your heart too weak or stiff to fill and pump efficiently." Source: http://www.mayoclinic.org/diseases-conditions/heart-failure/basics/definition/con-20029801

xvi **atrial fibrillation:** "Atrial fibrillation is an irregular and often rapid heart rate that commonly causes poor blood flow to the body. During atrial fibrillation, the heart's two upper chambers (the atria) beat chaotically and irregularly — out of coordination with the two lower chambers (the ventricles) of the heart. Atrial fibrillation symptoms often include heart palpitations, shortness of breath and weakness." Source: http://www.mayoclinic.org/diseases-conditions/atrial-fibrillation/home/ovc-20164923

xvii **heart ablation:** "Cardiac ablation is a procedure that can correct heart rhythm problems (arrhythmias). Ablation usually uses long, flexible tubes (catheters) inserted through a vein in your groin and threaded to your heart to correct structural problems in your heart that cause an arrhythmia. Cardiac ablation works by scarring or destroying tissue in your heart that triggers an abnormal heart rhythm. In some cases, ablation prevents abnormal electrical signals from traveling through your heart and, thus, stops the arrhythmia. Cardiac ablation is sometimes done through open-heart surgery, but it's often done using catheters, making the procedure less invasive and shortening recovery times." Source: http://www.mayoclinic.org/tests-procedures/cardiac-ablation/basics/definition/prc-20022642

xviii **ventricular tachycardia (v-tach):** "A type of heart rhythm disorder (arrhythmia) in which the lower chambers of your heart (ventricles) beat very quickly because of a problem in your heart's electrical system." Source: http://www.mayoclinic.org/diseases-conditions/ventricular-tachycardia/basics/definition/con-20036846

xix **heart transplant:** "A heart transplant is an operation in which a failing, diseased heart is replaced with a healthier, donor heart. Heart transplant is a treatment that's usually reserved for people who have tried medications or other surgeries, but their conditions haven't improved sufficiently. While a heart transplant is a major operation, your chance of survival is good, with appropriate follow-up care. When faced with a decision about having a heart transplant, know what to expect of the heart transplant process, the surgery itself, potential risks and follow-up care." Source: http://www.mayoclinic.org/tests-procedures/heart-transplant/basics/definition/prc-20014050

xx **transplant evaluation:** "Your evaluation may last one to two weeks and may include: physical examination; blood tests, including blood and tissue type analysis; imaging tests, including chest X-rays; cardiac catheterization; consultations with specialists in heart and blood vessel disease (cardiologists); transplant surgery; and social services. A team of doctors trained in heart and blood vessel disease (cardiologists), transplant surgery, infectious diseases, mental health conditions (psychiatrists) and other areas evaluate you to determine if you're eligible for a heart transplant. Doctors will explain what to expect after a heart transplant, including taking medications, lifestyle changes and other changes. Doctors will also discuss with you the risks and benefits of transplant surgery. If you're approved for a heart transplant, you'll be placed on a waiting list for a donor heart. You may be on a waiting list from a few days to several years. You'll need to manage your current health condition and have regular follow-up appointments with your doctor. While waiting for a donor heart, you'll need to remain in close contact with the transplant team and notify your transplant coordinator of any significant changes in your medical or social situation. You should be prepared to get to the hospital quickly after you receive notice that a donor heart is available. You may be eligible for a ventricular assist device or a total artificial heart to aid circulation while waiting for a heart transplant, or as a treatment instead of a heart transplant." Source: http://www.mayoclinic.org/departments-centers/transplant-center/heart-transplant/preparing/process

xxi **biventricular (BiV) ICD:** "Unlike a standard pacemaker, which stimulates only one side of your heart's main pumping chamber (the right ventricle), a biventricular pacemaker stimulates both the right and left ventricles to make the heart beat more efficiently. A special type of ICD — a combined biventricular pacemaker with ICD — can do the same thing. Biventricular pacing is particularly valuable for some people with heart failure whose hearts' electrical systems don't work normally." Source: http://www.mayoclinic.org/tests-

procedures/implantable-cardioverter-
defibrillator/basics/what-you-can-expect/prc-20015079

xxii **dobutamine IV drip:** "Dobutamine is used to help your
heart pump better by strengthening the heart muscle.
Dobutamine also improves blood flow and relieves symptoms
of heart failure." Source:
https://www.nlm.nih.gov/medlineplus/druginfo/meds/a682
861.html

xxiii **left ventricular assist device (LVAD):** "A left
ventricular assist device (LVAD) is implanted under your skin.
It helps pump blood from the left ventricle of your heart and
on to the rest of your body. A control unit and battery pack
are worn outside your body and are connected to the LVAD
through a port in your skin."
Source: http://www.mayoclinic.org/tests-
procedures/ventricular-assist-devices/multimedia/left-
ventricular-assist-device-lvad/img-20006714

xxiv **bleed everywhere:** Blood thinners are important to
prevent clotting of the blood, but an excess of the medication
may cause bleeding.

xxv **prednisone:** a corticosteroid drug. "Corticosteroids
mimic the effects of hormones your body produces naturally
in your adrenal glands, which sit on top of your kidneys.
When prescribed in doses that exceed your body's usual
levels, corticosteroids suppress inflammation. This can reduce
the signs and symptoms of inflammatory conditions, such as
arthritis and asthma. Corticosteroids also suppress your
immune system, which can help control conditions in which
your immune system mistakenly attacks its own tissues."

xxvi **eleven months:** Any type of surgery requires a significant for healing and return of function for the body. With transplantation the immune response has been pushed backward, and it takes longer to heal.

xxvii **quit smoking:** A patient cannot get an LVAD if he or she smokes because smoking has a negative impact on recovery and contributes to producing blockages in the coronary arteries of the heart.

xxviii **bicuspid rather than tricuspid:** The aortic valve normally has three flaps (leaflets) and is called tricuspid. Some people, however, are born with one that is bicuspid, having two flaps. As such, this valve is more narrow and subject to developing aortic stenosis. An excellent visual of heart with tricuspid and bicuspid valve can be seen at: http://www.mayoclinic.org/normal-heart-and-aortic-valve-stenosis/img-20007788

xxix **funny sounds coming from my heart my whole life:** Using a stethoscope, a doctor can detect the turbulence of blood flow passing through an abnormally narrow valve opening. This is called a heart murmur.

xxx **the Gibbs energy in thermal physics:** "In thermodynamics, the Gibbs free energy (IUPAC recommended name: Gibbs energy or Gibbs function; also known as free enthalpy to distinguish it from Helmholtz free energy) is a thermodynamic potential that can be used to calculate the maximum or reversible work that may be performed by a thermodynamic system at a constant temperature and pressure (isothermal, isobaric). Just as in mechanics, where the decrease in potential energy is defined as maximum useful work that can be performed, similarly different potentials have different meanings. The decrease in Gibbs free energy (kJ in SI units) is the maximum amount of non-expansion work that can be extracted from a thermodynamically closed system (one that can exchange heat and work with its surroundings, but not matter); this maximum can be attained only in a completely reversible process. When a system transforms reversibly from an initial state to a final state, the decrease in Gibbs free energy equals the work done by the system to its surroundings, minus the work of the pressure forces." Source: https://en.wikipedia.org/wiki/Gibbs_free_energy

xxxi **pleurisy:** "Pleurisy is a condition in which the pleura — a membrane consisting of a layer of tissue that lines the inner side of the chest cavity and a layer of tissue that surrounds the lungs — becomes inflamed. Also called pleuritis, pleurisy causes sharp chest pain (pleuritic pain) that worsens during breathing. A variety of underlying conditions can cause pleurisy. Treatment of pleurisy involves pain control and treating the underlying condition." Source: http://www.mayoclinic.org/diseases-conditions/pleurisy/basics/definition/con-20022338

xxxii **fibrillating:** "Atrial fibrillation is an irregular and often rapid heart rate that can increase your risk of stroke, heart failure and other heart-related complications. During atrial fibrillation, the heart's two upper chambers (the atria) beat chaotically and irregularly — out of coordination with the two lower chambers (the ventricles) of the heart. Atrial fibrillation symptoms often include heart palpitations, shortness of breath and weakness. ...Treatments for atrial fibrillation may include medications and other interventions to try to alter the heart's electrical system." Source: http://www.mayoclinic.org/diseases-conditions/atrial-fibrillation/home/ovc-20164923

xxxiii **angioplasty:** "Coronary angioplasty (AN-jee-o-plas-tee), also called percutaneous coronary intervention, is a procedure used to open clogged heart arteries. Angioplasty involves temporarily inserting and inflating a tiny balloon where your artery is clogged to help widen the artery." http://www.mayoclinic.org/tests-procedures/angioplasty/basics/definition/prc-20014401

xxxiv **blockages and calcifications:** The problem of blockages is a continuous ongoing manifestation of the slow, gradual production of fatty deposits, or *atheroma*, in the arteries.

xxxv **nitroglycerin pill:** Nitroglycerin works by relaxing blood vessels, thereby sending more blood and oxygen to the heart. An effect may include reduction in chest pain and light-headedness or dizziness.

xxxvi **monitoring tech:** An exercise technician is trained in monitoring a patient's heart rhythm during an exercise. This information helps guide the patient's exercise prescription.

xxxvii **Crestor:** "Crestor, a.k.a. Rosuvastatin, is used together with a proper diet to lower cholesterol and triglycerides (fats) in the blood. This medicine may help prevent or slow down medical problems, like atherosclerosis (hardening of the arteries), that are caused by fats clogging the blood vessels. It may also be used to prevent certain types of heart and blood vessel problems in patients with risk factors for heart problems. Rosuvastatin belongs to a group of medicines called HMG-CoA reductase inhibitors, or statins. It works by blocking an enzyme that is needed by the body to make cholesterol, so this reduces the amount of cholesterol in the blood." Source: http://www.mayoclinic.org/drugs-supplements/rosuvastatin-oral-route/description/drg-20065889

xxxviii **triple bypass:** Coronary bypass surgery is used to treat heart attacks or serious chest pain (angina) caused by blockages in the arteries that supply blood to the heart muscle. The surgeon attaches (grafts) a blood vessel taken from elsewhere in the body to the diseased heart artery, rerouting blood around the blockage in the same way a road detour re-routes traffic around road construction. A double, triple or quadruple bypass refers to the number of heart arteries that are bypassed." Source: http://www.secondscount.org/heart-condition-centers/info-detail-2/benefits-risks-of-coronary-bypass-surgery-2#.V9LoMvorK71

xxxix **LAD:** The left anterior descending artery in the heart.

xl **polymyalgia rheumatica:** "an inflammatory disorder that causes muscle pain and stiffness, especially in the shoulders." Source: http://www.mayoclinic.org/diseases-conditions/polymyalgia-rheumatica/basics/definition/con-20023162

xli **kinked right above the stent:** If coronary artery disease progresses after a stent is inserted, a subsequent blockage can develop just above the stent, causing a kink.

xlii **Prevent Heart Disease (PHD) Program:** a membership-based exercise program with options ranging from a completely self-guided program to one offering a customized exercise prescription targeting individual goals and periodic blood pressure, heart rate and oxygen saturation checks. Medical supervision is available for individuals at higher risk.

www.ingramcontent.com/pod-product-compliance
Lightning Source LLC
Chambersburg PA
CBHW020354290526
45785CB00005B/2277